Vegetarianism.

One Man's Views and Experiences

William McEwan

http://www.patonross.com/

Disclaimer:

This publication is designed for education purposes only,

and to share the Authors opinion and personal experiences concerning the subject matter covered.

The Author accepts no liability for damages arising from the abuse or misuse of the information contained within.

Thank You

Thank you for purchasing my book.
Please REVIEW it on Amazon –
Your feedback is important to me to assist
with the writing of my next book.

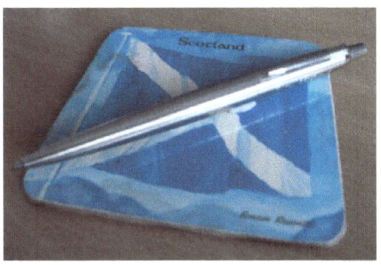

Thank you once again.

Forward.

Just recently, I found out that one of my granddaughters has decided to stop eating meat. My reaction is yes; it's one more of us and one less of them, well not really but at family barbeques or dinners I am usually the odd one out

As I am a non-meat eater, who also does not eat chicken, but I do eat fish, I am therefore not a true vegetarian.

Being part of a large family who are mostly meat eaters, it always gives me a lot of pleasure when another member of my family decides they are going to be a vegetarian,

This decided me to put together my own experiences gained over about thirty plus years as a non-meat eater.

This is not a diet book nor do I consider myself an authority on diet and nutrition. However, my experience and the knowledge gained from reading may help other people deciding to give up relying on dead animals as a food source.

Contents

Where does it all start

"If you don't eat your meat you'll not get any pudding" or so the saying goes; and it drums up a picture of a kid sitting at the table with a scowl on his face equally determined not to give in, but the parents usually win.

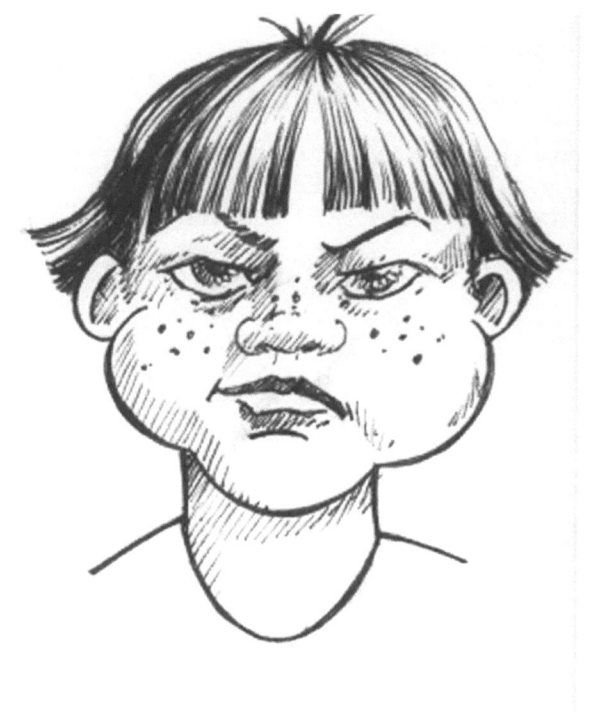

I have also heard parents tell their teenager who has decided to stop eating meat, "you will eat what is put on the table as long as you are under my roof".

Again, a clash of minds now I don't think this was a parent just being authoritarian, but cooking for the family may be cheaper and less trouble if one type of meal is prepared for everyone.

This does highlight the fact that parents, while believing that a child must have meat to survive, may cause a child who displays an aversion to meat to be tempted to eat the meat in order to get something sweet, or will eat meat just to please their parents.

Usually the child then becomes a meat eater into his or her adult life. Parents will then often accept the child eating potato chips, or pies and sweets as well as many other accepted foods that may then bring with them a host of health challenges.

For most people, meat eating is a lifetime diet; however, there are an increasing number of young adults and not so young who are adopting the vegetarian lifestyle.

The reasons they give are usually an aversion to animal cruelty, some for better health and others like me just because they do not like eating meat.

Non-meat eating is healthy, as long as you eat an alternative healthy diet, which sad to say is not always the case.

To explain what I mean is some people start the day with a cup of coffee and no breakfast.

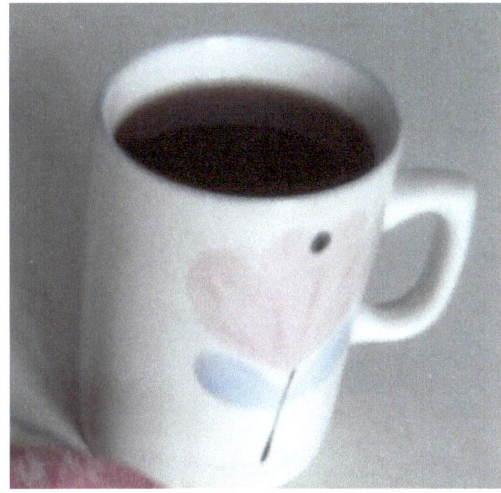

A couple of hours later another coffee accompanied by cakes, scones or muffins for morning break.

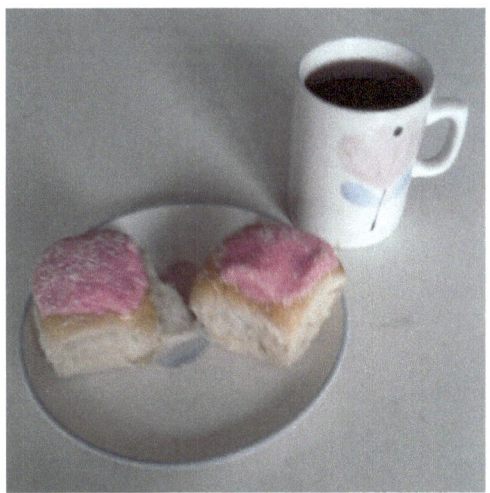

Lunch is a bag of potato chips and more coffee or soft drink

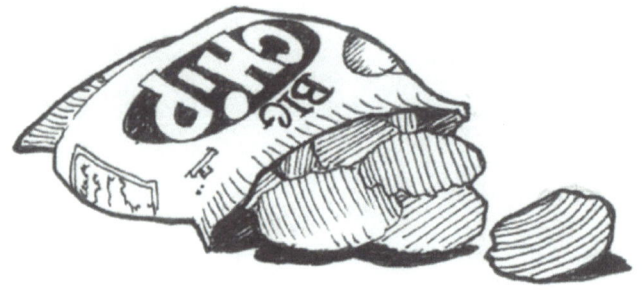

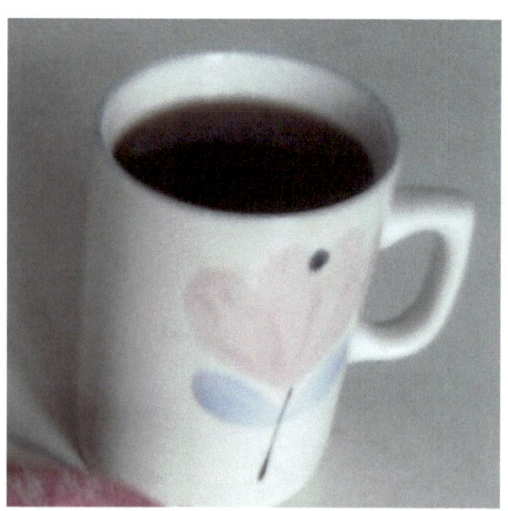

Then vegetarian pizza for an evening meal

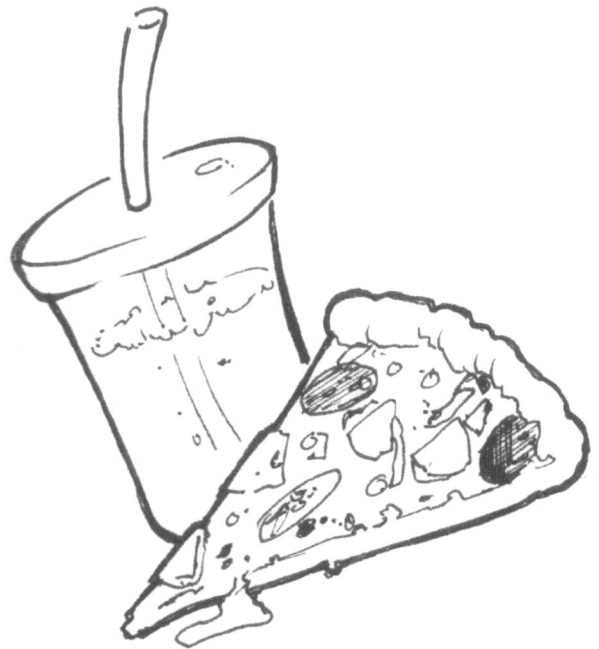

Although no meat eaten, the major problem is they were not eating anything nutritious, like fruit or vegetables.

Vegetables are essential for everyone particularly green vegetables and where possible raw.

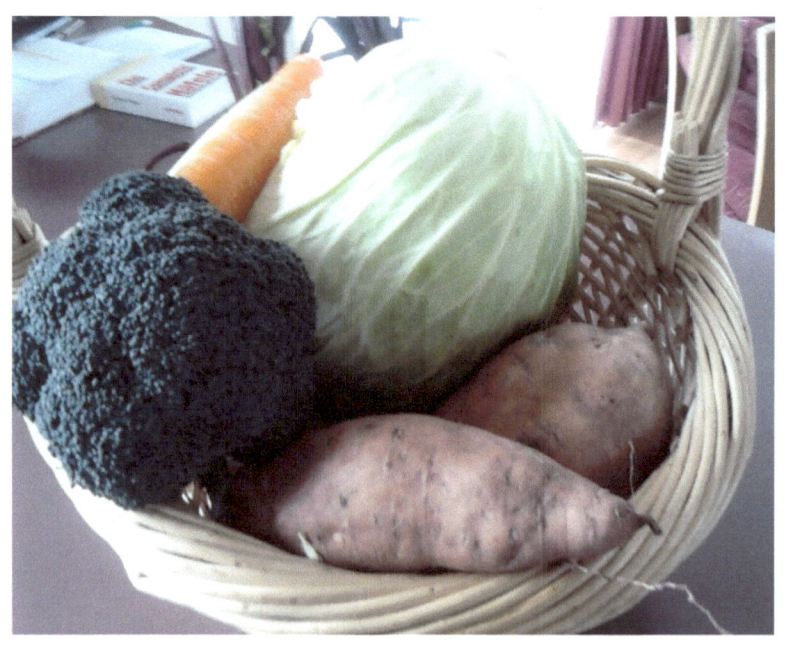

I recognised the fact that I was not an expert in nutrition, and for that reason, I adopted the use of multi vitamin and mineral supplements.

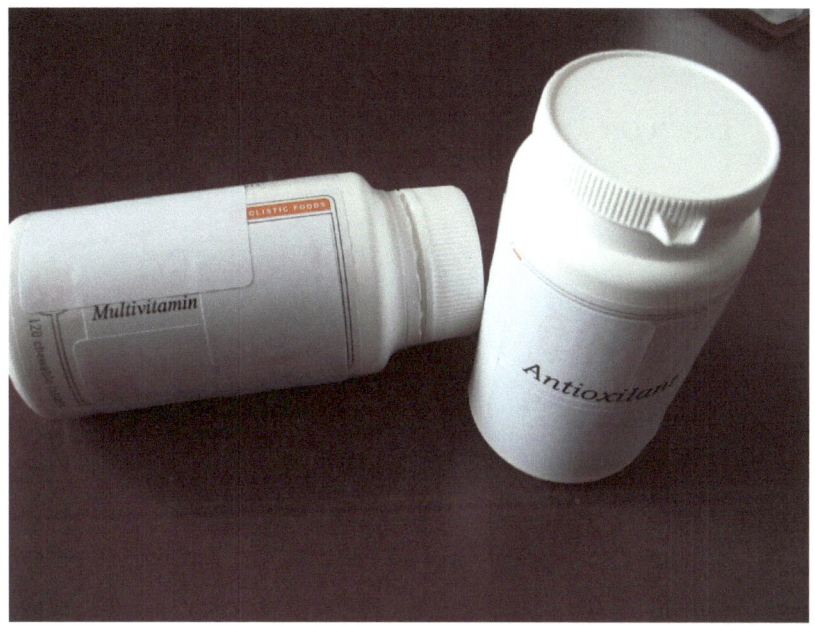

Believe me, after thirty plus years as a non-meat eater, and reading everything I could find about nutrition, and although I am now in my late seventies, I am still learning.

Don't be put off by the Naysayers

It is strange the reaction you get from some of your friends when you break away from the normal. Some made comments such as:

"Every vegetarian I know is extremely bad tempered"

"Did you know that when you pull up a lettuce it screams with pain?"

"Vegetarians always look half starved, thin and puny"

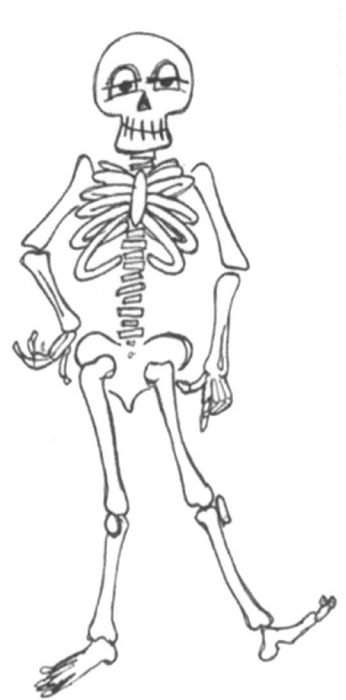

These were just some of the stupid comments made to me in an attempt to change my eating habits.

The best way to deal with these comments is just smile and nod, and let it wash over you as you carry on enjoying your food. The good news is that the negative comments eventually stop as the naysayers realise they are wasting their time.

From time to time, there are media items that could make you doubt the vegetarian lifestyle. I have always taken them with a pinch of salt and just think about who has the most to lose should more people start spending their money on vegetables.

Some concerned health professionals will point out that a vegetarian diet may be lacking in vitamin B12.and this of course is a concern.

However, fish and eggs, which I have always eaten, contribute to my need for Vitamin B12. If you don't eat fish or eggs the simple solution is to supplement many multi vitamin and mineral supplements contain vitamin B12.

Probably the best option is vitamin B12 tablets that dissolve under the tongue or a spray that can be used under the tongue.

In the 1970s when I first stopped eating meat, I soon found that non-meat eaters were not a chef's favourite customer. My very first experience of this was going out for a meal with a group of friends prior to a show. Everything on the menu contained meat, so I asked the waitress if I could have a meal without meat. She returned after speaking to the chef then informed me that he would provide a meatless meal.

Our entire group received their meals first, and when mine duly arrived, it turned out to be a plate with nothing but lettuce leaves and very little else.

I concluded that chefs were only trained to cook meat. Vegetables were only there to take up space on the plate, and cooking without meat was incomprehensible.

Fortunately, an increase in Asian restaurants has introduced vegetarian meals as part of their menus; in particular, Indian restaurants often have a vegetarian menu with a variety of very tasty and nutritious meals without meat that still have adequate protein.

Cafés have food cabinets and usually I find that with the exception of egg or cheese sandwiches and rolls the rest tend to have some form of meat even macaroni and cheese usually has bacon in it.

There are now vegetarian restaurants and cafes', but change has been slow despite a growing number of people that have stopped eating meat.

More Than One Type of Vegetarian:

Lacto-ovo-vegetarians eat both dairy products and eggs; this is the most common type of vegetarian diet

.

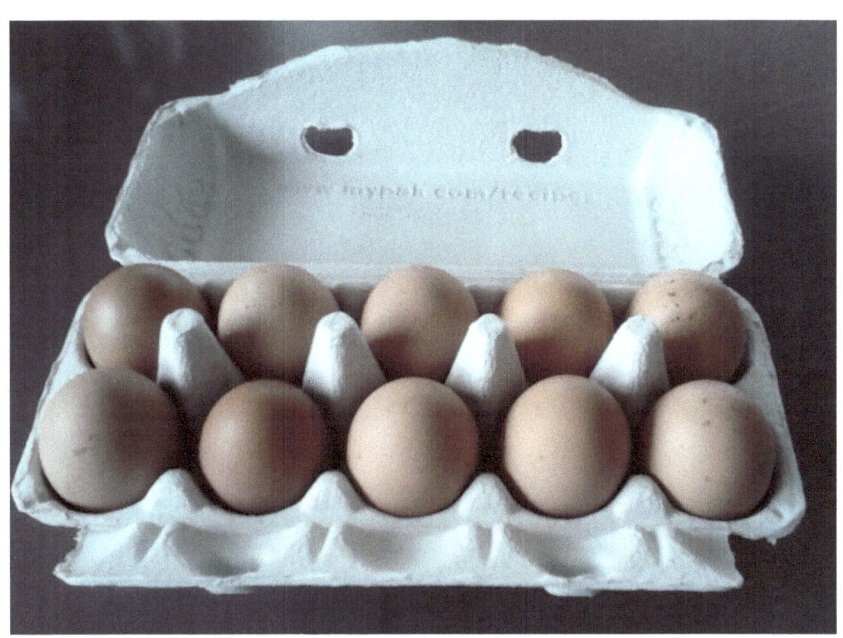

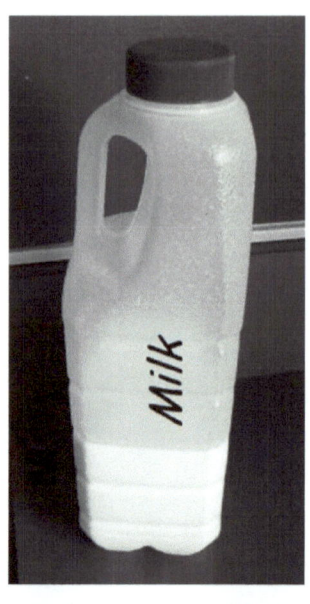

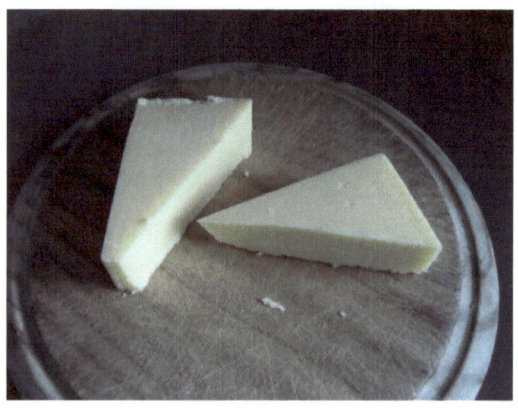

Lacto-vegetarians eat dairy products but avoid eggs.

Vegans do not eat dairy products, eggs, or any other products derived from animals.

Religious reasons:

Many people are vegetarian because of their religious beliefs for example: Hindus and Buddhists may choose to practice a vegetarian diet, also Jains who are pacifist to the extent they respect the right of every living creature. *(Jains wouldn't kill any living thing,)* Seventh day Adventists are recommended to avoid meat for health reasons.

There are a great many vegetarians past and present, many are our favourite actors and entertainers as well as sports personalities.

Proteins

Protein is not limited to meat in fact there are many excellent plant based proteins such as beans, nuts, flaxseed, pumpkin seed, sesame seed, sunflower seed, lentils and rice. Other sources of proteins that may be acceptable to vegetarians are:

Eggs: Many conscientious lacto-ovo vegetarians will only eat free-range eggs mainly due to objections to horrific treatment of hens because of intensive farming. It makes sense to believe a healthier chicken will lay healthier eggs.

Eggs are an excellent source of protein but also high in cholesterol, and it is believed this makes them a contributor to cardiovascular disease. However many health professionals now believe this is not true.

Sometimes when I feel I need a bit more protein I find that a plate of scrambled eggs does make me feel better.

Micro filtered or ultrafiltered whey is another complete protein.

Rice and lentils together provide a complete protein but it needs both.

Tofu is a well-recognised source of protein, however being a soy product there is some concern about the quality of soy as a very high percentage is genetically modified.

Low fat yogurt is a very good source of protein as is milk, cheese and multi-grain bread.

For The Good of our Health

Consuming animal fats and proteins has been linked to heart disease, as well as cancer of the colon and lung. It is also related to many debilitating conditions such as hypertension, obesity, kidney disease, diabetes and osteoporosis.

Milk, straight from the cow is very nutritious, unfortunately the milk supplied through normal retail outlets has been pasteurised and this destroys much of the nutritional value.

Cows milk is naturally meant for young calves and not good for humans. Strange when you think about it all animals get weaned off mother's milk and then feed with the adults, yet humans continue to drink the milk of other animals for the rest of their lives, maybe we need to grow up and learn to eat with the adults.

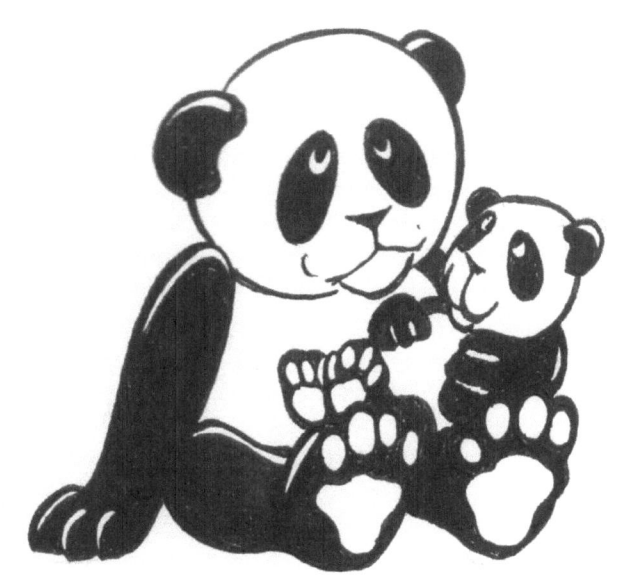

How do you cope with Various Diets?

In the past when my wife and I were invited out for a meal and we mentioned that I was a vegetarian our hosts would go into a tailspin. What could they possibly give me to eat? We would then explain just the same as every one else but without the meat, a simple solution.

Well not so, there was this pervading belief that that I must have some sort of substitute for meat. Fortunately, nowadays, close friends and family simply add an egg, some tuna or cheese, I am happy so; problem solved. In fact, a handful of walnuts or cashews would be a simple and inexpensive solution.

Up until about the 1960s it was taken for granted that except for a few individuals, everyone would eat meat and potatoes, not any more. In today's world, which is very cosmopolitan, food choices that were once considered obscure are now part of the mainstream.

The reasons why people choose special diets range from religious practices, ideological beliefs, allergies, special diets and food sensitivity's.

There are many various, life style eating philosophies around these days.

If you have to prepare meals for someone make sure you know if they have a particular requirement then it would pay to take time to research and understand the basic principles behind the diet.

Do the research.

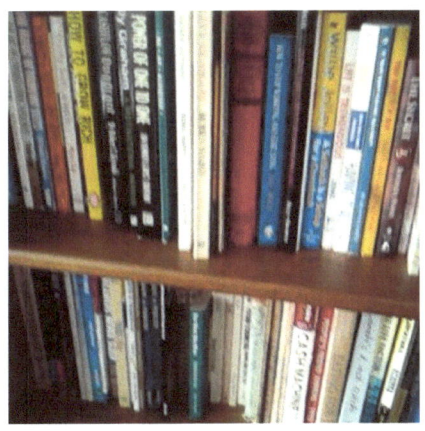

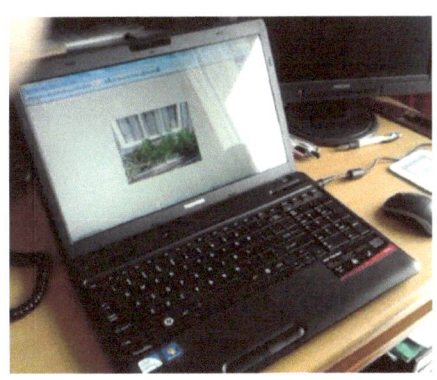

Allergies and Food Restrictions

When planning meals, or co-ordinating a function, preparing menus, always check if the guests have any allergies or food restrictions.

For example: Vegan, Muslim, Diabetic, Kosher, Lactose intolerant, Gluten free and egg free. Some may be allergic to potatoes or rice, peanuts, this is important as many allergies are life threatening.

Gaining knowledge in the fundamentals behind food allergies, restrictions and diets is not only beneficial for you when you play host, knowing the nutritional make up of various foods means that those with allergies will not have any nasty effects following eating and it is important to know what food is high or low in Carbohydrates, Minerals, Fats and Proteins.

Various religions and cultures may feel strongly about certain foods and food preparation.

Jews: Do not eat meat that has come from a pig.

Hindu: The cow is sacred to the Hindu and they do not eat beef and strict Hindus are vegetarians but there are some, who eat meat.

Sikh: Many Sikhs are vegetarians but in general, they don't have many strict rules about diet.

Buddhist: Strict Buddhists are vegetarians however because some live in India and others in China, available foods are different and their dishes may vary.

Meat Eating and the Environment

Animal agriculture takes a devastating toll on the earth. It is an inefficient way of producing food, since feed for farm animals requires land, water, fertilizer, and other resources that could otherwise have been used directly for producing human food.

Global warming is regarded a major threat to the planet and according to many climatologists there could be a limited time before we reach a stage where it could become irreversible. The motor car gets the blame but there is evidence that munching on dead animals is a more likely cause, not that it lets the car of the hook.

Some countries have major problems with water shortages yet it is known that we could save water by not eating meat, in fact by missing three or four hamburgers would save more water than not showering for six months. In terms of land wastage, it takes two hectares of land to feed one meat eater, yet one hectare would feed twenty people on a plant based diet.

Having said all that, I cannot claim any principle on my part for not eating meat I simply stopped because I don't like eating meat, but ok with fish so not a true vegetarian.

If you are thinking of trying a vegetarian lifestyle take advice from other vegetarians, join vegetarian organisations where you can have contact with other experienced vegetarians.

When I gave up eating meat, I knew very little about diet, or what nutrients I should pay attention to, I knew protein and vitamin B12 deficiencies could present a problem.

I learned later that because I ate fish and eggs that it meant I could be getting these nutrients. I found a book called "You Are What You Eat" by Victor Lindlahrs (1971 edition) and this had a profound effect on me at the time, and for years I used it for reference.

Benefit for Me

I can say from my own experience that stopping eating meat was a gigantic step in the right direction.

I experienced considerable health improvements despite the fact that I did nothing else to my diet to benefit my overall health.
For example: The annual coughs, colds, flu and tummy upset reduced dramatically. Bowel movements less of a challenge, and I felt a lot fitter to the extent that at the age of fifty five I trained for and ran a marathon, at the end of which I had a few aches but was not short of energy.

Over the years, I have collected many books on natural health and alternative therapies, which gives me a wealth of information, but one book, which outlines some major points that make a lot of sense, is called "Bragg Toxicless Diet" by Paul and Patricia Bragg. This book takes a back to basics approach in the sense it explains how we come to be eating the way we do.

I used to wonder why the human race eats the flesh of animals and birds, that unlike carnivorous animals, we are not designed to consume and digest animal flesh.

To try and find a solution that makes sense we need to think about how things were long before we could make a fire or even wear clothes.

Let's face it there must have been a time when we were not aware of how to make clothes, without clothes or the ability to start a fire to keep us warm we could only have survived in a climate that was warm all year round and at night, which would have been the tropics.

We would have been vulnerable to all predatory animals and totally dependant on vegetation such as fruit, nuts, seeds and roots for our food until such times we became aware of how to make a spear or club to hunt and kill small animals.

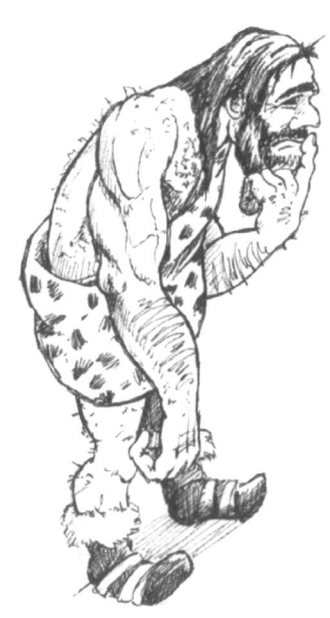

How long it took before we got to this stage one can only guess, whether it would have been thousands of years or millions of years either way it would seem we were designed eat fruit and vegetables.

However with necessity being the mother of invention and lifting our level of awareness there was a move away from tropical environments to cooler climates and a lack of the fruit that had been our staple diet. This changed the way we eat as we learned live by eating flesh of birds and animals. Evolution meant we also learned to make clothes, produce fire and survive colder climates.

These are my thoughts and seem to be the only explanation that makes sense to me. I have heard and read other explanations.

There are major benefits in a vegetarian lifestyle and what these benefits are no one will know until they try living without meat for about six months and feel the difference.

From the Ground Up

A major problem today is a lack of minerals in the soil in fact this was observed in the USA as far back as the 1930s and a document was presented to congress in 1936, 74th Congress, 2nd session.

This document showed concern over the deteriorating level of minerals in USA soils. We take minerals out of the soil, put very little back, and pay the price with health problems that can be traced back to nutritional deficiencies. If the minerals are not in the soil, then they are not in the food grown there and not in your diet.

In today's world, food supplementation is regarded as a necessity. Multi vitamin and minerals supplements help insure that you are getting the necessary nutrients. Be wary of synthetic supplements remember your body is organic and doesn't always respond well to synthetics.

Organic vegetables tend to cost more, but it doesn't need to be that way. A great source of good organic vegetables is to grow your own because you can prepare the soil and without good soil you get unfit vegetables and living on unfit food results in an unfit and unhealthy body if minerals are not in your soil they are not in your body where they are needed. If you have not got a garden you can grow them in pots or window boxes many people are doing this with great success.

The soil in our garden has a lot of clay and we have not had great success with our vegetables so we made up planter boxes and filled them with vegetable growing mix from the garden shop now things grow much better. They are fresh and taste so much better than those bought in the store.

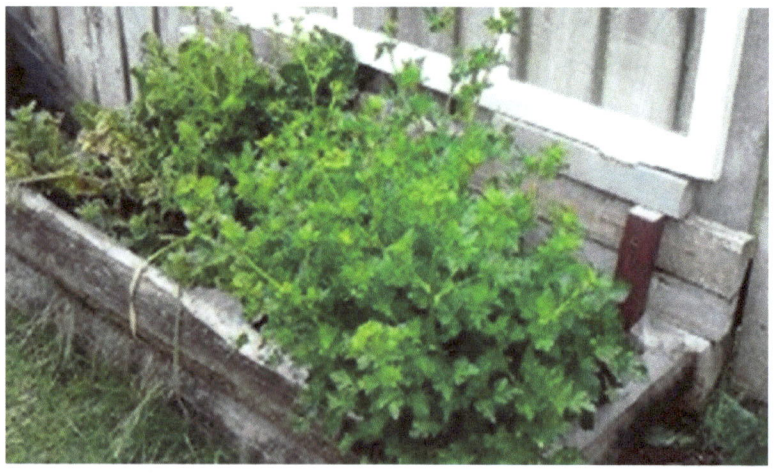

We also put all food scraps from the kitchen and garden waste in a large composting bin and periodically this compost is added to our planter boxes.

So now, if you are concerned about what is left for you to eat should you decide to give up meat then maybe the following list will give you some ideas.

Asparagus	Green beans
Avocados	Green peas
Beets	Kale
Bell Peppers	Leeks
Broccoli	Mushrooms
Brussels' sprouts	Mustard greens
Cabbage	Olives
Carrots	Onions
Celery	Potatoes
Collard greens	Lettuce
Cucumbers	Sea Vegetables
Eggplant	Spinach
Fennel	Squash
Garlic	Sweet potatoes
Swiss chards	Tomatoes
Turnip greens	Yams

Then there is also fish, eggs, cheese, bread, pasta, rice, quinoa, buckwheat, oats and nuts.

Fish provides an excellent source of omega 3 and protein. Eggs are probable the best source of protein of all foods and also an excellent source of tryptophan a precursor of serotonin which is very important for a good nights sleep.

Combining rice and lentils will also provide and excellent protein, also lentils are an excellent source of tryptophan.

Buckwheat is a protein food and cooking the groats makes beautiful porridge or can be soaked overnight and eaten raw they are also a very good source of tryptophan.

Similarly quinoa makes great porridge and high in tryptophan.

Oats cooked properly provide an excellent porridge, it is sugar free for all those trying to lose weight, if you need some flavouring my favourite solution is a sprinkle a little sea salt or Himalayan Red Salt:

I have used salt on my porridge since I was a child. Putting sugar on porridge is not a very good practice from a health point of view, and I feel it just spoils the whole experience of eating porridge.

In conclusion, is being a vegetarian worth the trouble? Well in my case, I have only experienced health benefits and have no regrets.

My advice is, decide why you want to stop eating meat, make a decision to change your lifestyle and in a few weeks, you will enjoy the result.

I know I did, as everything improved.

Just enjoy the food and ignore the naysayers.

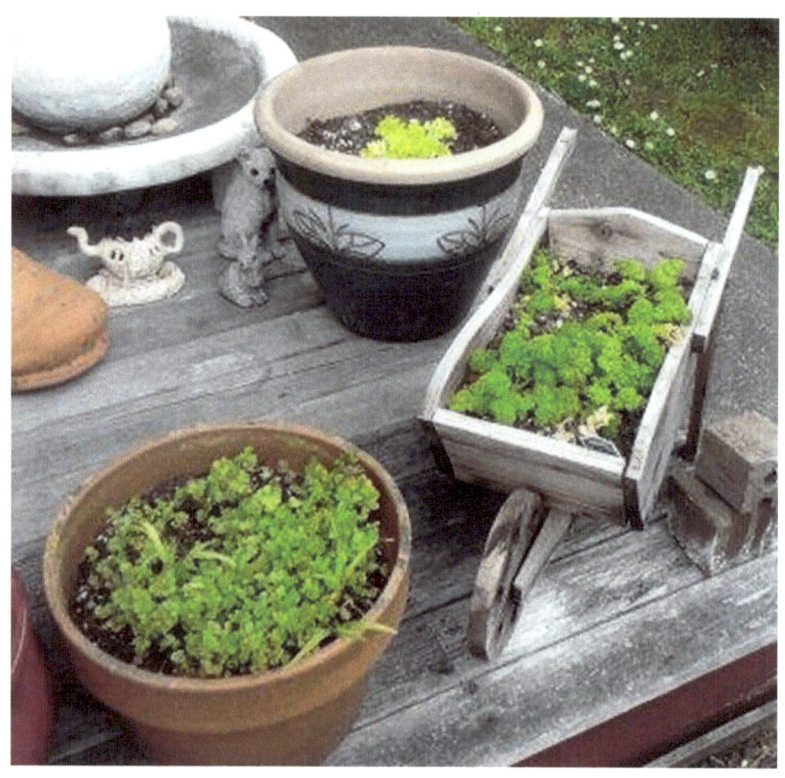

Other books by this Author.

A Reluctant Soldier

Short Stories from Rural Scotland

Graphics by courtesy of my son
davemcewan.com

and my wife Kate's Photographic skills.

Please take the time to visit our website

http://www.patonross.com/

www.ingramcontent.com/pod-product-compliance
Lightning Source LLC
Chambersburg PA
CBHW050858290526
45792CB00002B/641